Unlocking

Her

Pleasure

A comprehensive guide to Giving your Partner Mind Blowing Orgasms

Copyright © by Dr. Ann D. Foster 2022. All rights reserved.

TABLE OF CONTENT

INTRODUCTION

Giving your partner an orgasm is important for several reasons. First and foremost, it is bound to improve the emotional and physical connection between Partners. Thereby fostering a feeling of intimacy and closeness. Also, having an orgasm can improve one's physical and emotional well-being. Endorphins, endogenous painkillers, and mood enhancers are released during orgasms to aid in stress reduction and better sleep. This thorough manual provides different tips and methods for arousing different erogenous zones, combining naughty conversation and toys, as well as resolving problems like performance anxiety and mismatched libidos. But, it's crucial to keep in mind that achieving sexual pleasure is a process that requires time, perseverance, and work. In understanding and respecting your partner's unique wants and desires, as well as working together to explore and experiment in a safe and loving atmosphere, are the keys to unlocking your partner's pleasure leading to a more fulfilling and satisfying sexual relationship

CHAPTER **1**

UNDERSTANDING THE FEMALE ANATOMY

The Clitoris: What it is and how to stimulate it.

In female bodied individuals, the clitoris is a tiny extremely sensitive organ that is situated above the vaginal opening. It is a crucial component of the female sexual anatomy and the main source of sexual gratification for the majority of women. The clitoris is extremely sensitive to stimulation and touch because it has millions of nerve endings.

To Stimulate the Clitoris, There are several techniques you can try including:

1. Manual stimulation: You can gently massage or stroke the clitoris with your fingers in a circular or back-and-forth motion. Find the right pressure and speed by experimenting with them.

2. Oral stimulation: You can softly lick, suck, or kiss the clitoris using your mouth and tongue.

Once more, experiment with several methods and get your partner's opinion to see which feels the most comfortable.

3. Vibrator or sex toy stimulation: Several sex toys, such as vibrators, wand massagers, and suction toys, are made expressly to stimulate the clitoris. Try out various sorts and intensities to see what suits you best.

NOTA BENE

Let your spouse know what feels good and what doesn't through communicating with them. As every individual is unique, what works for one person may not work for another. Find what feels best for you by taking the time to explore and try different things. Also, keep in mind that the clitoris is a very sensitive organ, so be cautious and work up to more intense stimulation gradually.

The G-spot: Where it is and how to find it.

The front vaginal wall of those with female bodies contains the G-spot, an erogenous zone. It is a spongy tissue region that, when stimulated, is thought to be extremely sensitive and capable of producing strong sexual pleasure.

Yet it's vital to remember that not all females may have a G-spot or enjoy G-spot stimulation. It is preferable to initially become sexually aroused through foreplay to detect the G-spot because it tends to become more noticeable and simpler to locate when a person is sexually excited. When you become aroused, place one or two fingers inside the vagina and curl them upward until they are two to three inches from the belly button. The G-spot should have the texture of a slightly elevated or rough tissue region.

NOTA BENE

a)Let your spouse know what feels good and what doesn't through communicating with them. Try out various postures and strategies to see what works best for you. Some people discover that using a sex object made for G-spot stimulation, like a curved dildo or a G-spot vibrator, can be beneficial.

b)Keep in mind that it's quite common for not everyone to have a G-spot or feel pleasure from G-spot stimulation. Instead of placing pressure on yourself to locate a specific location or to experience a specific style of orgasm,

The most crucial thing is to put your attention on enjoying and communicating with your partner.

Other erogenous zones of the body

Numerous additional parts of the body can be extremely sensitive and receptive to sexual stimulation, while the clitoris and G-spot are two of the most well-known erogenous zones. Enhancing your partner's sexual pleasure and intimacy can be enjoyable and thrilling by exploring these other erogenous zones. Some erogenous areas to think about investigating include:

1. Lips: Lips may be quite sensual and delightful to kiss and nibble on.

2. Ears: Lightly nibbling or caressing the earlobes, as well as murmuring loving or lustful phrases, can be quite exciting.

3. Neck: For many people, the neck is a very sensitive place. Intense pleasure can be produced by kissing, nibbling, or even just gently blowing on the neck.

4. Nipples: The nipples have a lot of nerve endings and can be very sensitive to touch. Try out various forms of touch, like licking, sucking, and gentle pinching.

5. Inner thighs: For many people, the inner thighs can be an erogenous zone since they are extremely sensitive. Gently massaging or kissing the inner thighs can be incredibly exciting.

6. Feet: The feet have many nerve endings and can be particularly sensitive to touch. A foot massage or mild tickling can be pleasurable.

NOTA BENE

Keep in mind that every person has a unique body, so what works for one person might not work for another. It's crucial to talk to your spouse and experiment with different body parts to discover what makes you feel happy. Increased sexual pleasure and intimacy can result from taking the time to explore and experiment.

CHAPTER 2

BUILDING SEXUAL TENSION

The importance of foreplay

Foreplay is an essential component of sexual intimacy that involves any sexual behavior that occurs before sexual penetration. It's an opportunity to establish arousal and intimacy between lovers, and it can considerably boost sexual pleasure and satisfaction for both partners. These are some reasons why foreplay is important:

1. **Builds arousal:** Foreplay helps to develop arousal and anticipation for sexual activity, which can enhance sexual enjoyment and lead to more intense and fulfilling orgasms.

2. **Enhances intimacy:** Participating in foreplay can help lovers feel more connected and intimate. It's an opportunity to explore each other's bodies and wants and to speak about what feels good and what doesn't.

3. Improves lubrication: Foreplay helps to promote natural lubrication in the vagina, which can make sexual penetration more pleasant for both partners.

4. Reduces stress and anxiety: Participating in sexual activity can be a stress-relieving activity that helps to reduce anxiety and increase emotions of relaxation and well-being.

5. Allows for experimentation: Foreplay is the perfect opportunity to explore with different touch, stimulation, and sexual activities. It's a chance to explore each other's bodies and discover new methods to enjoy pleasure together.

NOTA BENE

Remember, foreplay is not a one-size-fits-all activity. Speaking with your spouse and finding what feels enjoyable for both of you is crucial. Take the time to explore and experiment, and don't hesitate to attempt new things. The most important thing is to focus on pleasure and closeness with your spouse.

How to develop sexual tension in your relationship

Creating sexual tension with your spouse may be a fun and exciting approach to enhance closeness and pleasure. These are some ways for increasing sexual tension:

1)Great Anticipation: Send sexy texts or messages throughout the day, letting your lover know that you're thinking about them and looking forward to becoming intimate later. Create anticipation by hinting at what you'd want to do together.

2)Physical touch: Touch your lover in intimate ways throughout the day, such as kissing their neck or holding their hand. This might develop excitement and anticipation for more personal touch later on.

3)Eye contact: Establish eye contact with your partner in a way that expresses your desire and interest. Eye contact may be a strong method to establish sexual tension and intimacy.

4)Try new things: Try new sexual activities or positions that you haven't done before.

This can bring excitement to your sexual experiences and generate anticipation for what's to come.

4)Slow things down: Take your time with foreplay and build arousal steadily. This can prepare one in anticipation and heighten pleasure when you finally do become intimate.

5)Use your words: Speak with your spouse about what you find attractive about them and what you're looking forward to in your sexual experiences together. Verbalizing desire can be a powerful method to develop sexual tension and connection.

NOTA BENE

Remember, developing sexual tension is all about creating anticipation, excitement, and connection with your partner. Talk openly and explore different approaches to find what works for you and your spouse.

The Use of Dirty talk and other techniques to increase Arousal

Using dirty words to stoke excitement before sexual activity can be entertaining and thrilling.

It's crucial to discuss this form of sexual communication with your spouse and make sure you both feel at ease with it. Here are some pointers on using sex cues and other strategies to pique interest:

1. Begin gradually: Start by saying things like, "I adore the way you feel," or "you make me feel so good." This can help to gradually increase arousal and foster anticipation.

2. Pay attention to your Partner's Response: To determine whether your spouse is enjoying the obscene chat, pay attention to their reaction and verbal clues. It's crucial to respect their boundaries and cease approaching them if they appear uneasy or uninterested.

3. Be Specific: When expressing what you desire or what you find alluring about your partner, use words or phrases that are explicit. Intimacy and a sense of connection between lovers may result from this.

4. Use your voice: Generate distinct moods and feelings by experimenting with different tones and loudness of your voice. Many people can be immensely aroused by soft whispers or moans.

5. Employ non-verbal communication: To complement your dirty words and improve the sexual experience, use body language like touching, kissing, or eye contact.

6. Experiment with other techniques: To increase arousal and pleasure during sexual activity, try other techniques like using sex toys, incorporating role-play, or experimenting with different positions.

NOTA BENE

Always be mindful that sexual communication should be respectful, consensual, and centered on mutual enjoyment. Openly discuss your preferences with your partner, and be willing to try new things and learn new things together.

Chapter 3:

TECHNIQUES FOR GIVING HER AN ORGASM

Oral Sex: Tips and Tricks for Pleasuring Her With Your Mouth

When performed properly, oral sex can be a very pleasurable experience for both partners. Here are some pointers for mouth- gratification with her:

1. Communicate: Before you begin, find out what your partner enjoys and dislikes. Because everyone has different preferences, it's critical to understand what appeals to her.

2. Take it slow. Begin by using light, teasing touches with your tongue or lips. Use gentle suction and explore her body slowly, building arousal over time.

3. Employ your hands: Stimulate her clitoris or other erogenous zones using your hands as part of your oral sex technique. You can also explore her body and direct your mouth with your hands.

4. Experiment with various techniques to see which ones feel most comfortable for her. For example, change the pressure, speed, or positioning of your mouth and tongue.

5. Pay attention to her responses: To determine what is working and what is not, observe your partner's body language and pay attention to her vocal cues. To increase arousal and increase pleasure, adjust your technique as necessary.

6. Maintain a steady rhythm: Once you find a method that works, keep it up to help arousal rise and orgasm occur.

7. Don't forget the clitoris: For many women, the clitoris can be a major source of pleasure. It is a highly sensitive area. Try out various methods, such as using your tongue, lips, or fingers to stimulate the clitoris.

NOTA BENE

To find what works for you and your partner, it's important to experiment and communicate openly because everyone has different preferences. Don't forget to put your partner's comfort and enjoyment first, and don't be shy about seeking advice or feedback along the way.

Fingering: How to entice her with your fingers

When done properly, fingering can give women a great deal of pleasure. Here are some pointers on how to stimulate her with your fingers:

1. Communicate: Before you begin, find out what your partner enjoys and dislikes. Because everyone has different preferences, it's critical to understand what appeals to her.

2. Get ready: Trim your nails and make sure your hands are clean. To make the experience more enjoyable and smooth, lubricant your fingers.

3. Begin slowly: Start by giving your fingers a few light, teaser touches. Slowly increase your arousal by slowly exploring her body.

4. Use your fingers to stimulate the G-spot: a highly sensitive region on the upper wall of the vagina, by inserting one or two fingers into her vagina and moving them in a come-hither motion.

5. Experiment with various techniques to find what feels comfortable for her: For example, change the pressure, speed, or position of your fingers.

6. Pay attention to her responses: To determine what is working and what is not, observe your partner's body language and pay attention to her vocal cues. To increase arousal and increase pleasure, adjust your technique as necessary.

7. Use your thumb: While your fingers are inside her, use your thumb to irritate her clitoris. For many women, the clitoris can be a significant source of pleasure because it is a very sensitive area.

8. Maintain a steady rhythm: To help increase arousal and trigger an orgasm once you've found a technique that works.

NOTA BENE

To find what works for you and your partner, it's important to experiment and communicate openly because everyone has different preferences. Don't forget to put your partner's comfort and enjoyment first, and don't be shy about seeking advice or feedback along the way.

Toys: Incorporating toys into Foreplay

To enhance your partner's and your own sexual experiences, consider using sex toys. Here are some tips on incorporating sex toys into your play.

1)The importance of communication is strongly advised so always have a discussion with your spouse about your interests and comfort levels before introducing sex toys. Talk about any issues or limitations you may have.

2)Start small and easy: like with a vibrating bullet or a small dildo, if you or your partner are new to sex toys. This can make using toys together more comfortable for you both.

3 Explore together: Spend some time using the toys to explore each other's bodies. Try out various positions and methods to see what works best for you and your partner.

4. Utilize lubricant: Using sex toys can be made more delightful and comfortable by using lubricant. Choose a lubricant that is water-based and appropriate for the toy you are using.

5. Clean your toys: To stop the transmission of bacteria, keep your sex toys clean and well-maintained. Observe the cleaning and storing recommendations provided by the manufacturer.

6. Have an open mind: Be willing to explore new things and play with various toys. You might learn novel ways to enjoy each other's company that you had never even considered.

7. Don't be scared to ask for assistance: If you need assistance using a toy or want to learn more about a specific product, don't be reluctant to do so. To get the most out of your toys, several sex toy retailers provide information and tips.

NOTA BENE

Always keep in mind that using sex toys should be fun and consensual for both couples. Find what works for you both by taking the time to explore options and speak honestly with one another.

CHAPTER 4

COMMUNICATING WITH YOUR PARTNER

The importance of Communication in Sexual Relationships

Every part of a successful sexual relationship requires communication. Here are some justifications for why communication is crucial:

1)Recognizing one another's needs: Each has unique sexual preferences as well as desires and limitations. Partners can better comprehend one another's requirements and guarantee that they are both pleased by open and honest communication.

2)Communicating your thoughts and feelings regarding sex with your spouse: This will help you two become more intimate and trusting of one another. This may result in a more intense emotional bond and satisfying sexual encounter.

3)Conflict resolution: Sexual troubles and disagreements can occur in every relationship. Partners can work together to identify answers and maintain a healthy and pleasant sex life by discussing openly and addressing difficulties as they come up.

4)Seeking new experiences: Effective communication can aid couples in exploring new sexual possibilities. By discussing fantasies and desires, partners can experiment with new activities that are mutually satisfying.

5)Ensuring Safety: To ensure that both partners are protected against sexually transmitted diseases (STIs) and unintended pregnancies, it is crucial to communicate about sexual health and safety.

NOTA BENE

Always remember that communication should be respectful and non-judgmental. It's critical to provide a secure and welcoming environment where partners may speak candidly and openly. Partners can create a stronger, more fulfilling sexual relationship by putting communication first.

How to talk to your partner about their desires and preferences

Even though it might be a sensitive topic, discussing your partner's preferences and desires is crucial to developing a strong sexual relationship. Here are some tips to help you go about the discussion.

1)Choose the right time and place: Choose a time and location where you and your partner may speak to each other privately and without interruption. Make sure you are both comfortable and at ease.

2)Start with something encouraging: Express your desire to learn more about your partner's sexual desires and preferences. Let them know you're concerned about their requirements and wish to meet your wants as well.

3)Ask Open-ended questions: Ask your partner open-ended questions to get their opinions and feelings. Avoid asking questions that have a straightforward "yes" or "no" response.

4)Be Non-Judgemental: Listen to your spouse without passing judgment and refrain from critiquing or discounting their views.

Recall that every person has distinct and legitimate sexual preferences.

5)Share your feelings and thoughts: Moreover, express your ideas and sentiments around sex. This might encourage a more direct and sincere conversation.

6)Be patient: it could take some time for your partner to open up to you about their preferences and desires. Be understanding and patient.

7)Respect boundaries: If your partner is reluctant to provide specific details, don't press the matter. The subject can always be brought up again in the future.

NOTA BENE

The foundation of a successful sexual relationship is communication. You and your spouse can develop a closer bond and have a happier sex life together by being upfront and honest about your needs and preferences.

Tips On Giving and Receiving Feedback

Giving and receiving feedback is an important aspect of any relationship, including sexual relationships. Here are some Tips for efficiently providing and accepting feedback:

Giving Feedback

1)Be precise: Be specific when expressing your opinions by stating what you like and don't like. So your partner will be able to clearly see what they can do to get better as a result of this.

2)Instead of using "you" statements, use "I" statements: Say "I would prefer it if you did it this way," for instance, rather than "You did this improperly." By doing this, you can make your partner feel less defensive and more open to your advice.

3)Focus on the positive: When providing criticism, start by highlighting what your partner did well as a result, they will become more self-assured and open to receiving constructive criticism.

4)Be kind: Be sympathetic and kind when providing feedback. Keep in mind that your partner is probably trying their best and wants to win your approval.

Receiving Feedback

1)Active listening: Actively listen when getting critique, and make an effort to comprehend your partner's viewpoint. Do not respond defensively or discount their suggestions.

2)If you're not sure of what your partner is saying, ask for clarification: This can aid in your understanding of their criticism and suggestions for improvement.

3)Do not personalize it: Keep in mind that criticism is not a personal affront. It's a chance for you to develop and get better as a partner.

4)Saying Thanks: Even though it's challenging to hear, thank your partner for their input. Tell them that you value their openness and that you'll make an effort to improve.

NOTA BENE

Keep in mind that both offering and accepting feedback require practice.

Unlocking Her Pleasure

You can establish a secure and encouraging environment where the two of you may develop together by being open and honest with your partner.

CHAPTER **5**

OVERCOMING COMMON CHALLENGES

Dealing with performance anxiety.

Performance anxiety is a common issue that can affect both men and women during sexual activity. It can result in a variety of symptoms, such as difficulty getting or maintaining an erection, premature ejaculation, or difficulty reaching orgasm. Here are some tips for dealing with performance anxiety:

1)Relax: Breathe deeply and work to relax your body. Anxiety can be lessened by relaxation techniques like yoga or meditation.

2)Putting pleasure first Instead of stressing about your performance: Concentrate on the joy you are feeling. Try diverse methods of sexual gratification with your spouse, such as oral sex or utilizing toys.

3)Speak to your partner about your anxiety and collaborate to find a solution: This can foster intimacy and lessen the pressure to do well.

4)Self-care is the act of looking after oneself: To do this, maintain a good diet, get enough sleep, and exercise frequently.

5)Consider obtaining professional assistance from a therapist or counselor if your anxiety persists or is affecting your sexual life: You can learn from them how to handle your nervousness and enhance your sexual performance.

NOTA BENE

Remember that a lot of people suffer from performance anxiety. You can have a healthy and enjoyable sex life by taking steps to lessen worry and being transparent with your partner.

Addressing mismatched libidos

Having a mismatched libido, where one partner has a higher sex drive than the other, can be a common issue in relationships. Here are some tips for addressing mismatched libidos:

1)Open communication: Discuss your sex drive with your spouse and how it affects your connection. Be open and sincere about your wants and desires, and listen to your partner's perspective as well.

2)Find a Common ground: Find a compromise that benefits both of you by working together. This can entail striking a balance concerning frequency or looking into alternative forms of intimacy.

3)Explore nonsexual intimacy: Keep in mind that closeness is much more than just sex. Try to make other connections with your partner, such as kissing, embracing, or cuddling.

4)Consult a professional: Consider consulting a therapist or counselor for assistance if your relationship is being negatively affected by your mismatched libido or is experiencing substantial stress as a result. They can assist you in identifying the underlying reasons for the problem and provide you with the tools and techniques you need to enhance your sexual relationship.

5)Keep calm: It can require patience and time to address mismatched libidos. Always remember to show your partner compassion and understanding, and be prepared to collaborate with them to find a solution that benefits both of you.

How to handle sexual dysfunction

Sexual dysfunction can affect both men and women and can include a range of issues such as difficulty getting or maintaining an erection, premature ejaculation, difficulty reaching orgasm, and low libido. Here are some tips for handling sexual dysfunction:

1)Speaking with your partner: To address sexual dysfunction, communication is essential. Be upfront and honest with your partner when discussing the problem, and work together to find a solution that benefits both of you.

2)Address any underlying medical conditions: An underlying medical condition like diabetes, heart disease, or hormone imbalances may be the root of some sexual dysfunction. To find out whether any medical disorders are causing the issue, consult your doctor.

3)Consult a professional: You can manage sexual dysfunction with the aid of the tools and strategies a therapist or counselor can give you. They can provide you with ways to address any psychological or emotional aspects that may be causing the problem as well as assistance in identifying any such variables.

4)Consult medication: Medication may occasionally be useful in the treatment of sexual dysfunction. See your doctor about your alternatives and whether they would be the best ones for you.

5)Test out other approaches: To find what works best for you and your partner, try out a few various positions and tactics. This can enhance sexual enjoyment and lessen anxiety.

NOTA BENE

Recall that sexual dysfunction is a widespread problem that affects lots of people. You may come up with a solution that works for both of you by being willing to explore various approaches, obtaining professional assistance, and having open communication with one another.

Your sexual relationship may always be improved, but it takes work and dedication on both partners' parts. Here are some suggestions for enhancing your sexual connection moving forward:

a)Stay in touch frequently: A healthy sexual relationship requires open communication regularly. Continue discussing your wants and requirements with your partner while also paying attention to their opinions and preferences.

b)New endeavors: To keep things interesting and thrilling in the bedroom, experiment with various approaches, positions, and imaginations. Be curious and open to experimenting with novel concepts and feelings.

c)Taking care of yourself: A fulfilling sexual relationship depends on good physical and mental health. Take good care of yourself by eating healthily, working out frequently, getting adequate sleep, and controlling your stress levels.

e)Make time for intimacy: Make intimacy a priority in your relationship and arrange a time for it in your busy schedule. This can be done by scheduling a regular date night or weekend getaway or by simply scheduling a quick daily cuddle or kiss.

f)Continue to learn: To continue learning about new techniques to enhance your sexual connection, read books, go to workshops, or ask other couples about their experiences.

To improve your sexual connection, keep in mind that both partners must put in effort and devotion. You may continue to improve your sexual relationship and deepen your connection with your spouse by communicating frequently, trying new things, taking care of yourself, scheduling time for intimacy, and be open to learning.

Conclusion:

Better understanding of your Partner's needs and desires requires good communication. This will deepen the emotional connection between both parties, increasing intimacy that will open the door to more frequent and higher quality sex. It's crucial to keep in mind that achieving sexual pleasure is a process that requires time, perseverance, and work.